Pedro Paulo Dias Soares
Leonardo Caixeta
George Silva Junior

Evolution from Bipolar Affective Disorder to Dementia

Pedro Paulo Dias Soares
Leonardo Caixeta
George Silva Junior

Evolution from Bipolar Affective Disorder to Dementia

Impact of treatment and length of bipolar disorder, types and number of crises on dementia outcome

ScienciaScripts

Imprint
Any brand names and product names mentioned in this book are subject to trademark, brand or patent protection and are trademarks or registered trademarks of their respective holders. The use of brand names, product names, common names, trade names, product descriptions etc. even without a particular marking in this work is in no way to be construed to mean that such names may be regarded as unrestricted in respect of trademark and brand protection legislation and could thus be used by anyone.

Cover image: www.ingimage.com

This book is a translation from the original published under ISBN 978-613-9-76497-6.

Publisher:
Sciencia Scripts
is a trademark of
Dodo Books Indian Ocean Ltd. and OmniScriptum S.R.L publishing group

120 High Road, East Finchley, London, N2 9ED, United Kingdom
Str. Armeneasca 28/1, office 1, Chisinau MD-2012, Republic of Moldova, Europe
Printed at: see last page
ISBN: 978-620-6-44071-0

SUMMARY

Introduction/Objectives: To discuss the relationship between bipolar affective disorder and dementia, specifically patients diagnosed with bipolar affective disorder and dementia. **Methods:** Survey of data on the treatment of bipolar disorder and dementia syndrome, the impact of lithium on treatment, the relationship between length of bipolar disorder, the number and type of seizures and progression to dementia outcome. **Results**: The predominant dementia in the overall sample is corticobasal dementia, 46.9 per cent (table 2). Lithium is the third main medication used for mood stabilisation, being used by 8.5% of the sample, or 24.4% of the people who used some medication. The effect of lithium is not significantly different from the effect of the other drugs in improving the patient's condition. It was found that the patient's improvement was not associated with the total number of crises. Among those with predominantly mania, only 33.3 per cent showed some improvement, a significantly lower proportion than the proportion of improvement in those without mania, 77.9 per cent. **Conclusions:** The use of lithium was not superior to other mood stabilisers when treating patients with dementia and mood disorders. In this study, there was no evidence of a proportional link between the number of bipolar disorder crises and a worse dementia prognosis. Bipolar patients with a prevalence of manic crises have a worse recovery in dementia treatment than others. In other words, the variable "type of crisis" had more influence than the variable "duration of crises" or "number of crises".

Keywords: Bipolar disorder; Dementia; Mania; Lithium

SUMMARY

CHAPTER 1

INTRODUCTION

Knowing the relationship between bipolar affective disorder and the dementia process can deepen our understanding of both nosologies, as well as the intricate relationships that generate a causal link between the two. It is essential to re-discuss a psychiatric illness (bipolar affective disorder) which, if under-treated or untreated, can trigger progressive and irreversible dementia. Finally, rediscussing this requires evaluating the forms of treatment, the pathophysiological types of bipolar disorder, as well as the efficacy of lithium compared to other stabilisers.

The discussion about bipolar affective disorder in the development of dementia is important and focussed on prevention, suicide and costs. It is also essential to know how Bipolar Disorder and the dementia process are related, preventing the dementia outcome in Bipolar Affective Disorder.

Bipolar disorders are characterised by their phasic, episodic and chronic nature, the latter being similar to other mental disorders. These episodes occur in a time-limited manner, with periods of remission, with the patient remaining euthymic and with minimal or absent psychopathological alterations (AZORIN, J. M. *et al*, 2012).

The classic subtypes of bipolar disorder in psychiatric literature are: Type I Bipolar Disorder, with mild to severe depressive episodes, interspersed with phases of normality and well-characterised manic phases, and Type II Bipolar Disorder, with mild to severe depressive episodes, interspersed with periods of normality and followed by hypomanic phases (AKISKAL, H. S.; PINTO, O.,1999).

Bipolar disorder is still one of the most complex diseases to treat in all of medicine and can be considered resistant in patients who have difficulty achieving recovery. Only through a thorough psychiatric and clinical investigation in order to identify comorbidities can the situation of resistance be better explained (CAIXETA, 2006b).

In dementias, on the other hand, there is a progressive impoverishment and depletion of all psychic processes, mainly cognitive but also affective. In the most typical cases, such as Alzheimer's dementia (AD), memory loss is mainly concentrated in recent memory and fixation. There is also progressive neglect of personal hygiene, clothing, eating, physiological activities and toileting (DALGALARRONDO, 2008).

There may be a predilection, in the case of dementias that arise after years of bipolar disorder evolution, for less typical forms of dementia, called Non-Alzheimer's Dementia, with behavioural manifestations predominating, at least in the early stages of the dementia process, as is the case with Fronto-Temporal Lobar Degeneration (CAIXETA, 2016).

In dementia syndromes, the clinical aspects are the most relevant: memory loss, loss of multiple cognitive functions, changes in executive functions, personality changes, insidious and progressive course, presence of diffuse changes in brain tissue, normal level of consciousness and associated psychiatric symptoms (paranoid ideas, depression, anxiety, hallucinations, delusions and heteroaggression (KESSING, L V; NILSSON, F M, 2003).

The differential diagnosis of dementias includes pseudodementia caused by depressive disorder, *delirium* and mental retardation. The most frequent aetiological causes of dementia are: Alzheimer's disease, vascular dementia, dementia caused by Lewy bodies, subcortical dementia, frontotemporal dementias and mixed dementias (focal or localised psycho-organic syndromes: amnestic syndromes, frontal syndromes, temporal syndromes and parietal syndromes (NG, B *et al,* 2008).

The most common causes of dementia in individuals over the age of 65 are (1) Alzheimer's disease (2) vascular dementia and (3) vascular dementia and Alzheimer's type. Other diseases that account for around 10 per cent of the total include dementia with Lewy bodies; Pick's diseases; frontotemporal dementias; normal pressure hydrocephalus; alcoholic dementia; infectious dementia and Parkinson's disease (CAIXETA, 2008).

The treatment of dementia includes the management of cognitive decline and neuropsychiatric (behavioural) symptoms. Studies suggest that more than half of patients with dementia have two behavioural symptoms, making it necessary to carefully assess the drugs used and the enzyme system involved in their metabolism to avoid drug interactions and intoxication (CAIXETA, 2010).

Older people with bipolar disorder are classified into two categories. The first, called late-onset bipolar disorder, is characterised by the presence of the first episode only after the age of 50. In the other category, early-onset bipolar disorder is defined by the presence of the first episode before the age of 50, the two situations being quite distinct and important (CAIXETA *et al*, 2016).

The theory that better control of bipolar disorder by means of mood stabilisers reduces or slows down the development of dementias is well-founded, so much so that other researchers have demonstrated a prophylactic effect of lithium on the executive function of cognition (CAIXETA *et al*, 2016).

Mood disorders have been correlated with cognitive alterations since ancient times in medicine. Although there was no distinction between the concepts, because at that time only the concept of Melancholia was used, but cognitive deficits were already described as part of this condition by Hippocrates. Then, new concepts from the beginning of the 20th century - such as dementia, as it is understood today, separate from the concept of Bipolar Disorder - made it possible to more clearly correlate cognitive symptoms with affective conditions (CAIXETA, 2012).

Also according to the researcher mentioned below, the research of Alexopoulos (1993) led to the notion of reversible dementia in late-life depression and raised many questions about the nature of the relationship between mood disorders and dementia. The difficulty in identifying Depression when comorbid in various works supports the possibility of a common underlying pathophysiology for Depression and Vascular Dementia, although there are still many controversial points on the subject (SILVA JR., 2015).

Some propose the concept of a "depression-dementia spectrum" or even an "Alzheimer's disease dementia-depression spectrum" (SILVA JR., 2015). On the other hand, there are still many divergent findings and little research into the relationship between Bipolar Disorder, with its various clinical forms, and the different types of dementia (CAIXETA, 2006a).

CHAPTER 2

LITERATURE REVIEW

Bipolar disorder has been associated with cognitive decline and some studies investigating the risk of dementia and death in older people with bipolar disorder have concluded that bipolar disorder in senile age is associated with an increased risk of dementia (designated as greater neurocognitive impairment in the Diagnostic and Statistical Manual of Mental Disorders, Fifth Edition) and premature death (VALIENGO *et al,* 2016). Bipolar disorder is a chronic psychiatric illness characterised by fluctuations in mood, with a relapsing and remitting course (RUBINO *et al*, 2017).

There may be a predilection, in the case of dementias that arise after years of bipolar disorder, for less typical forms of dementia, with behavioural manifestations predominating, at least in the early stages of the dementia process, as is the case with Fronto-Temporal Lobar Degeneration (PAPAZACHARIAS *et al*, 2017).

In terms of psychopathology, Bipolar Disorder can hypothetically be divided into two large groups: patients who evolve "without" cognitive loss and those "with" cognitive loss. In the latter, cognitive loss can be associated with the final evolution to dementia in at least three ways (SILVA JR., 2015).

In a first subgroup would be patients with increased risk factors due to the behavioural changes that make up the clinical picture of bipolar disorder; in a second subgroup would be patients whose association would occur by chance between two different diseases; and in a third subgroup would be patients in whom bipolar disorder would lead to the wear and tear of brain circuits and cognitive reserve due to some form of neurotoxicity that would be intrinsic to it: Vesanic Dementia (SILVA JR., 2015).

The second subgroup would be patients whose association between two different diseases would occur by chance. Although this possibility always exists, there seems to be a greater chance of dementia among TB sufferers than would be supported by the casual association, since the risk of dementia increases by between 6% and 13% with each acute episode of bipolar disorder (SILVAJR.,2015).

In the third subgroup, the patients would represent the clinical phenotype of a neurodegeneration induced by the pathophysiology of bipolar disorder, in other words, a form of dementia intrinsic to it, Vesicular Dementia, as many pre-Kraepelian psychiatrists called it and which historically came to be considered a phase in the natural history of Bipolar Disorder, when there was little to offer in the way of specific treatment for bipolar disorder (SILVA JR., 2015).

Bipolar disorder has been associated with cognitive decline and has been researched, with the following findings: while bipolar disorder is local and functional, with the dementia process, neurological damage becomes regional and diffuse (SILVA JR., 2015).

The risk of dementia and death in the elderly was investigated, with the following results: bipolar disorder in the elderly implies a higher risk of suicide, a higher risk of dementia and lower performance on cognitive tests (RISE, 2016).

On the other hand, some epidemiological studies have shown that depression and bipolar disorder are risk factors for dementia and various aspects such as diet, exercise, lithium evaluation, vascular disease and the use of glucocorticoids have been investigated in order to identify preventive factors for dementia. The main conclusions were that suffering is a major risk factor in bipolar disorder and that prevention could be achieved through diet, exercise, lithium use, treatment of vascular disease and glucocorticoids (BABAH, 2016).

Other researchers have verified the need for specific clinical care, increased training and education for the elderly, in a sample of 37,768 patients aged 65-85 years, and found that bipolar disorder in the elderly increases the risk of dementia, but that the risk is lower in patients who have had bipolar disorder for less than 5 years. They also reported increased mortality in these patients from causes such as pneumonia or influenza, as well as diseases of the digestive system, suicide and accidents (ALMEIDA *et al*, 2016).

Regarding the discussion on the impact of lithium when compared to other mood stabilisers for the treatment of dementia, the study points out that valproic acid is widely used to treat patients with bipolar disorder, however, it has adverse effects on cognitive function (TSAI *et al,* 2016).

On the other hand, according to the following study, lithium is the first-choice medication, as it promotes a reduction in the risk of dementia in patients with bipolar disorder, and patients using lithium had negative cognitive tests; it was also found that the use of lithium can reduce the development of cognitive impairment in the elderly (CAIXETA *et al*, 2016).

Finally, with regard to the association between the length of illness, the number of seizures in patients with bipolar disorder and the interference of these variables in the evolution of dementia, there are studies that rule out this association in Alzheimer's dementia (CAIXETA, 2012), for example, on the grounds that cognitive deterioration in bipolar disorder is not associated with the classic pathophysiological mechanisms observed in Alzheimer's disease, i.e. the deposition of amyloid and hyperphosphorylation of the tau protein associated with microtubules (FORLENZA *et al,* 2016).

The association between frontotemporal dementia (non-Alzheimer's type) and bipolar disorder was also discussed, exploring a case study of a patient who arrived at the neuropsychiatry service with inappropriate laughter, hyperthymia and was finally diagnosed with dementia.

It was pointed out in another reference that many patients considered to have vesicular dementia at the beginning of the 20th century could actually be diagnosed with fronto-temporal dementia due to their affective symptoms, especially in cases of late-onset bipolar affective disorder. He emphasised that many patients with Fronto-Temporal Dementia, in a disinhibition syndrome, easily meet the criteria of the ICD-10 (World Health Organisation, 1993) and the DSM-V (American Psychiatry Association, 1994) for a manic episode. Despite this apparent difficulty, he emphasised the differentiating criteria between the mania of bipolar affective disorder and the disinhibition of a patient with FTD (CAIXETA, 2010).

This study was based on a rare sample (patients diagnosed with dementia and bipolar affective disorder simultaneously) whose small number, 130 patients, poses statistical challenges. On the other hand, some studies have indicated that samples of this type are small in research carried out in developing countries, when compared to the age pyramid of highly developed countries (PICINNI *et al*, 2015).

An early stage of behavioural variant frontotemporal dementia (bvFTD) usually shows a mixture of behavioural disturbances and personality changes that prevent a differential diagnosis from elderly bipolar disorder (BD), making this process very challenging (BAEZ *et al*, 2017).

A history of bipolar disorder is associated with a significantly higher risk of dementia in older adults (DINIZ *et al*, 2017).

However, although many anatomopathological lesions have been described, as well as various clinical, cognitive and functional deficits, these associations are still at the research stage (VASCONCELOS-MORENO *et al,* 2016), with studies leading to divergent conclusions, pointing to the need for further research (GAMA *et al*, 2013) into the clinical and neuropathological evolution of Bipolar Disorder and its correlation with its longitudinal course (KOTZIAN *et al*, 2016) (neuroprogression).

CHAPTER 3

OBJECTIVES

3.1.PRIMARY OBJECTIVE

To analyse the relationship between the variables of Bipolar Affective Disorder and its outcome in Dementia Syndromes.

3.2.SECONDARY OBJECTIVES

Evaluate the treatment history for patients with bipolar affective disorder recorded in the database.

To investigate whether different types of psychopharmacological treatment interfere with the progression of bipolar disorder to dementia syndrome.

To find out whether there is a relationship between the duration of bipolar disorder and progression to dementia.

Establish the relationship between the number of bipolar crises and progression to dementia.

CHAPTER 4

METHODOLOGY

The sample evaluated is one hundred and thirty (130) members of the Dementia and Bipolar Affective Disorder Database. It will consist of all (100 per cent) of the records that make up the Database (130 records, i.e. n=130), with no need for a sample extraction process, since all the records have been searched, i.e. the research sample coincides with the Database sample.

The database consists of 130 coded records, selected from a universe of 600 medical records from the Dementia Outpatient Clinic at HC-FMUFG and the Memory and Behaviour Institute - IMC, both in Goiânia, GO (SILVA JÚNIOR, GMN, 2015). The experimental procedure consists of searching this database.

The database was searched for relationships, frequencies and data that would allow comparisons to be made that would directly or indirectly answer the following problems listed above: What impact does the treatment of bipolar affective disorder have on progression to dementia? Is there a difference between the impact of lithium compared to other mood stabilisers? Do the duration of bipolar disorder and the number of crises interfere with the evolution of dementia? A correlation was made between bipolar affective disorder and the dementia syndrome, specifically those topics that include the role of mood stabilisers, the preventive capacity of lithium and the influence of crises in triggering the dementia process.

The statistical analysis used the following statistical tests: Chi-square, Mann-Whitney test and Fisher's exact test.

The study design is observational, cross-sectional and retrospective: the surveys in the Database cover data collected from the medical records from which the Database was built, in 2014 and 2015. These records are chronological and portray the evolution of the clinical condition of the 130 cases studied over time, such as an evolutionary record that contains notes in the medical records dating back to 1997.

The data collected was analysed using IBM SPSS (*Statistical Package for the Social Science*), version 22.0.

To characterise the sample and carry out a descriptive analysis of the behaviour of the variables, the data was summarised by calculating the descriptive statistics mean, median, minimum, maximum, range, standard deviation (SD), coefficient of variation (CV), proportions of interest, graphs and simple frequency distributions and cross-tabulations.

The distribution of frequencies in classes of a quantitative variable was obtained by determining the number of classes using the Sturges Formula.

In the inferential analysis, statistical significance tests were carried out to analyse whether the differences found between the distributions and statistics (proportions and averages) of different subgroups were significant. Two complementary proportions were compared using the Binomial Test. In the Inferential Analysis of the Distributions of Qualitative Variables, the significance of the association between two variables, or the difference between the distributions of the proportions, was investigated using the Chi-squared test and, when the Chi-squared test proved inconclusive, Fisher's Exact test was used. The Odds Ratio (OR) was the measure used to express any risk to be assessed. The significance of the OR was assessed by the confidence interval of the OR, at the 95% confidence level, which cannot contain the value 1 to confirm the significance of the OR, which would mean that the two subgroups had the same chance of presenting the characteristic or outcome being assessed.

In the Inferential Analysis of Quantitative Variables, the hypothesis of normality of distribution was verified by the Kolmogorov-Smirnov (KS) and Shapiro-Wilk (SW) tests. The distribution was considered normal only if both tests did not reject the hypothesis of normal distribution. When comparing two independent groups, the comparison was made using the Student's t-test. As in all the analyses of this type carried out in this study, at least one of the groups did not show a normal distribution in the variable being tested, the comparison of the two independent groups was made using the Mann-Whitney non-parametric test.

All discussions were carried out considering a maximum significance level of 5% (0.05), i.e. the following decision rule was adopted in the tests: rejection of the null hypothesis whenever the p-value associated with the test was less than 0.05. In the tests that provided asymptotic and exact p-values, the exact p-values were taken into account. Details of the statistical methodology can be found in the aforementioned literature review (FAVERO, 2009; MEDRONHO,2009).

It is important to emphasise that the study was retrospective and not prospective. As such, the retrospective study facilitates memory bias, which jeopardises the statistical result, because if the study were continuous, the number of patient crises would be reported with greater accuracy.

CHAPTER 5

RESULTS AND DISCUSSION

5.1.RESULTS AND DISCUSSION OF THE SOCIAL PROFILE

The sample resulted in 130 patients diagnosed with Dementia and Bipolar Affective Disorder, of which 78 were female (60.0%) and 52 were male (40.0%). The binomial test shows a significant difference between these proportions (p-value=0.028) and leads us to conclude that in the population of patients with dementia and bipolar affective disorder, there is a significant predominance of women.

The distribution of all the variables characterising the sample profile can be seen in Table 1. The typical patient was female (60.0%), lived in an urban area (at least 57.7% of patients), was married (at least 36.2% of patients) and white (at least 61.5%). The most frequent age groups were 64 to 72 years (at least 20.8% of patients), 80 to 88 years (at least 23.8% of patients) and 72 to 80 years (at least 20.8% of patients). The most frequent educational levels were 1 to 4 years of schooling (at least 15.4% of patients) and 4 to 7 years of schooling (at least 16.2% of patients), as shown in Table 1:

Table 1: Social Profile of the Sample

Variable	Frequency n	% Gross
Sex		
Female	78	60,0%
Male	**52**	**40,0%**
Home		
Not registered	27	20,8%
Urban Area	**75**	**57,7%**
Rural Area	26	20,0%
Both	2	1,5%
Marital status		
Not registered	40	30,8%
Single	3	2,3%
Married	**47**	**36,2%**
Widowed	31	23,8%
Separated/Divorced/Divorced	9	6,9%
Ethnicity		
Not Registered	33	25,4%
White	**80**	**61,5%**
Black	2	1,5%
Mestizo	14	1,1%

Yellow	1	0,8%
Age (years)		
Not registered	4	3,1%
40 |-48 years	1	0,8%
48 - 56 years	5	3,8%
56 - 64 years	10	7,7%
64 |- 72 years	**32**	**24,6%**
72 |- 80 years old	**27**	**20,8%**
80 |- 88 years old	**31**	**23,8%**
88 |- 96 years old	17	13,1%
96 | 104 years old	3	2,3%
Schooling (Years of Study)		
Not registered	42	32,3%
Illiterate	8	6,2%
1 to 4 years	**20**	**15,4%**
4 to 7 years	**21**	**16,2%**
7 to 10 years	6	4,6%
10 to 13 years	16	12,3%
13 to 16 years old	10	7,7%
16 to 19 years old	4	3,1%
19 to 22 years old	3	2,3%

Table 2 shows the main statistics for the distribution of age and years of schooling for the overall sample and by gender. Overall, the patients ranged in age from 43 to 101 years, which resulted in a mean of 76.2 years, a median of 76.8 years and a standard deviation of 11.4 years, with a coefficient of variation of 0.154, showing low variability between the patients' ages. The p-values of the normality tests lead to the rejection of the hypothesis of normality of the age distribution in the female and male subgroups. Therefore, the ages of patients in the female and male subgroups were compared using the Mann-Whitney test, which resulted in a p-value of 0.551.

As for the patients' schooling, the sample was very heterogeneous. Overall, the patients had between 0 and 22 years of schooling, which resulted in a mean of 7.2 years, a median of 5.0 years and a standard deviation of 5.8 years, with a coefficient of variation of 0.80, showing very high variability between the patients' schooling. The p-values of the normality tests lead to the rejection of the normality hypothesis for the distribution of years of schooling in the female and male subgroups. Therefore, the distributions of the patients' years of schooling in the female and male subgroups were compared using the Mann-Whitney test, which resulted in a p-value of 0.120.

Table 2; Patients' age and years of schooling

Statistics	Subgroup		
	Global	Female	Male
Age (years)			
Average	76,2	76,2	76,1
Median	76,8	78,9	74,3
Standard Deviation	11,4	11,7	10,9
Minimum	43	43	59
Maximum	101	96	101
Range	57,2	52,5	41,6

C.V	0,15	0,15	0,14
p-value of K.S test	0,200	0,200	0,034
p-value of SW test	0,418	0,070	0,016
p-value of the MW test comparing the age of patients in the male and female subgroups		0,551	
Schooling (Years of Study)			
Average	7,2	6,5	8,2
Median	5,0	4,0	6,0
Standard Deviation	5,8	5,8	5,7
Minimum	0	0	0
Maximum	22	22	21
Range	22	22	21
C.V	0,80	0,89	0,70
p-value of K.S test	0,000	0,000	0,000
p-value of SW test	0,000	0,000	0,007
p-value of the MW test comparing the schooling of patients in the male and female subgroups		0,120	

Table 3 shows the prevalence of psychological comorbidities among the patients in the sample. All the patients had at least one psychiatric comorbidity and the most prevalent comorbidities were Bipolar Disorder Grade I (BIT) with 61 cases, 46.9% of the patients, and Mixed Disorder with 50 cases, 38.5% of the patients. The distribution of frequencies between those who treat and do not treat psychiatric comorbidity, overall, and for each comorbidity can also be seen in Table 4. The incidence of treatment of psychic comorbidity is 44.6 per cent (58 out of 130 patients) and 55.4 per cent of patients did not treat psychic comorbidity. There was no significant difference between these proportions (p-value = 0.254, Binomial test). Analysing by comorbidity, it can be seen that for almost all comorbidities there is no considerable difference between the proportions of patients who treated the comorbidity and the proportion of patients who did not treat the comorbidity. The main differences can be seen for TBII, for which the majority of patients were not treated (70.8 per cent), and for Cyclothymia, for which 100 per cent of patients were not treated.

We investigated whether the treatment of psychological comorbidity was associated with the patient's gender. In the male subgroup, the incidence of treatment for psychological comorbidities was 46.6 per cent (27 out of 52 patients); in the female subgroup, the incidence of treatment for psychological comorbidities was 53.4 per cent (31 out of 78 patients). The chi-squared test showed no significant difference between these proportions (p-value=0.171).

We investigated whether the treatment of the psychological comorbidity had any association with the patient's age. Patients who treated their comorbidities had an average age of 70.5 years, d.p=9.8 years and a median of 70.3 years, while those who did not treat their comorbidities had an average age of 71.9 years, d.p=11.9 years and a median of 75.8 years. The Mann-Whitney test showed no significant difference between the age distributions of the two groups (p-value=0.493).

We investigated whether the treatment of the psychological comorbidity had any association with the patient's schooling. Patients who treated their comorbidities had an average of 8.1 years of schooling, a median of 6.5 years of schooling and a standard deviation of 6.5 years of schooling; and those who did not treat their comorbidities had an average of 6.8, a median of 5 years of schooling and a standard deviation of 5.1 years of schooling. The Mann-Whitney test showed no significant difference between the schooling distributions of the two groups (p-value=0.805).

Table 3: Prevalence of psychological comorbidities among patients,

Comorbidity	n	Prevalence in the Sample	Did not treat comorbidity		Treating comorbidity	
Global	130	100,0%	72	55,4%	58	44,6%
Dementia and Disorders Bipolar I	61	46,9%	36	59,8%	25	41,0%
Dementia and Mixed Bipolar Disorder	50	38,5%	24	48,0%	26	52,0%
Dementia and Disorders Bipolar VI	45	34,6%	19	42,2%	26	57,8%
Dementia and Disorders Bipolar II	24	18,5%	17	70,8%	7	29,2%
Dementia and Bipolar Disorder with prevalent bouts of Mania	8	6,2%	4	50,0%	4	50,0%
Dementia and bipolar disorder with preceding hypomanic attacks	8	6,2%	4	50,0%	4	50,0%
Dementia and bipolar disorder with prevalent cyclothymia	10	7,6%	7	100,0%	0	0,0%
Dementia and bipolar disorder with bouts of depression	1	0,8%	0	0,0%	1	100,0%

Table 4 shows the main statistics for the Age of Onset of Psychic Comorbidity, the time of comorbidity until inclusion, and the number of crises, overall and for each comorbidity. The comorbidities that are discovered earliest are Depression, TBI, TBII and Cyclothymia, diagnosed on average before the age of 40. Consequently, these comorbidities have the longest average comorbidity times until inclusion in the study. Mixed Disorder, Hypomania, Mania and Cyclothymia a are diagnosed, on average, over the age of 60; consequently, these comorbidities have the lowest mean comorbidity times until inclusion in the study.

The number of seizures varied greatly in the sample, from 1 to 41, with an average of 4.4 seizures per patient. The comorbidity with the highest average number of seizures was TBI and TBII. In all the comorbidities, the number of seizures had high variability, except for the patients with Cyclothymia, which had no variability and all the patients with this comorbidity only had one seizure.

We investigated whether the treatment of the psychological comorbidity had any association with the age at the onset of the comorbidity. Patients who treated their comorbidities discovered their comorbidities at a mean age of 55.4 years, d.p=18.5 years and a median of 59 years; and those who did not treat their comorbidities discovered their comorbidities at a mean age of 49.5 years, d.p=19.6 years and a median of 47.1 years. The Mann-Whitney test showed no significant difference between the age distributions at the onset of comorbidity in the two groups (p-value=0.117).

We investigated whether the treatment of psychological comorbidity had any association with the time of comorbidity until inclusion. Patients who treated their comorbidities had an average of 20.4 years of comorbidity, a standard deviation of 16.9 and a median of 13.5 years of comorbidity; and those who did not treat their comorbidities had an average of 27.4 years of comorbidity, a standard deviation of 19.2 and a median of 22.0 years of comorbidity. The Mann-Whitney test showed a significant difference between the distributions of time with comorbidity in the two groups (p-value=0.048).

We investigated whether the treatment of the psychological comorbidity had any association with the number of crises. Patients who treated their comorbidities had an average of 4.8 seizures, a standard deviation of 5.5 seizures and a median of 4 seizures; those who did not treat their comorbidities had an average of 4.0 seizures, a standard deviation of 2.8 seizures and a median of 3 seizures. The Mann-Whitney test showed no significant difference between the distributions of the number of seizures between the two groups (p-value=0.424).

Of the 58 patients who reported treating their mental comorbidities, only 45 had their medication recorded. For the majority of these 45 patients, 62.2% (28 patients) used only 1 medication. 20.0% (9 patients) used two medications in combination, 13.3% (6 patients) used 3 medications in combination. One patient (2.2%) used four different medicines and another patient (2.2%) used 6 different medicines to treat his psychological comorbidity.

Table 4: Age at onset of psychological comorbidity and time of comorbidity until inclusion, overall and for each comorbidity.

Comorbidity	Age of onset of comorbidity			Comorbidity time until inclusion			Number of Crises		
	Average	DP	CV	Average	DP	CV	Average	DP	CV
Global	51,3	20,5	0,4	25,2	18,9	0,75	4,4	4,2	0,95
Dementia and TBI	37,5	12,9	0,34	36,6	15,8	0,43	5,9	5,4	0,91
Dementia and	> 60 years	nc	nc	9,5	9,0	0,95	2,5	1,5	0,61

Mixed TBI									
Dementia and TBVI	73,5	8,5	0,11	8,4	6,7	0,80	2,7	1,5	0,57
Dementia and TBII	38,3	10,5	0,27	30,1	18,8	0,63	3,6	3,0	0,82
Dementia and TBI Mania	74,9	7,8	0,11	5,2	4,8	0,91	2,6	1,4	0,54
Dementia and bipolar disorder with seizures	68,5	4,7	0,07	9,4	6,3	0,67			
Hypomania							2,6	1,1	0,40
Dementia and Bipolar Disorder with	38,6	12,3	0,32	24,0	22,5	0,94			
Cyclothymia							1,0	0,0	0,00
Dementia and bipolar disorder with bouts of depression	From a young age	-	-	>50 years	nc	nc	4	nc	nc

Table 5 shows the frequency distribution of the medication used to treat psychological comorbidities. The most commonly used drugs are Olanzapine (11.5% of the sample and 33.3% of those who used some medication) and Quetiapine (10.8% of the sample, 31.3% of those who used some medication). Lithium is the third main medication used for mood stabilisation, being used by 8.5% of the sample, or 24.4% of those who were using some medication.

Table 5: Frequency distribution of medication used to treat psychological comorbidities

Medication used for mood stabilisation	Frequency	Percentage in the Sample	Percentage of those who had registered medication
Olanzapine	15	11,5%	33,3%
Quetiapine	14	10,8%	31,1%
Lithium	11	8,5%	24,4%
Valproate Sodium/Divalproate	8	6,2%	17,8%
Carbamazepine	8	6,2%	17,8%
Lamotrigine	5	3,8%	11,1%
Risperidone	5	3,8%	11,1%
Oxcarbamazepine	4	3,1%	8,9%
Gabapentin	2	1,5%	4,4%
Clonazepan	1	0,8%	2,2%
Mirtazapine	1	0,8%	2,2%

Table 6 shows the frequency distribution of types of dementia. The most prevalent dementias are Corticobasal, Frontotemporal, Alzheimer's and Vascular.

Table 6: Frequency of Types of Dementia

	Percentage in the Sample
Corticobasal	34,6%
Fronto-temporal	30,0%
Alzheimer's	23,1%
Vascular	21,5%

Lewy bodies	10,0%
Dem SOE	3,1%
Pick's disease	2,3%
Progressive Supranuclear Palsy	1,5%
Systemic lupus erythematosus	0,8%
Huntington's disease	0,8%
Hydrocephalus of Normal Pressure	0,8%

The medication used to treat dementia is very varied. The most commonly used drugs and their frequency can be seen in Figure 1:

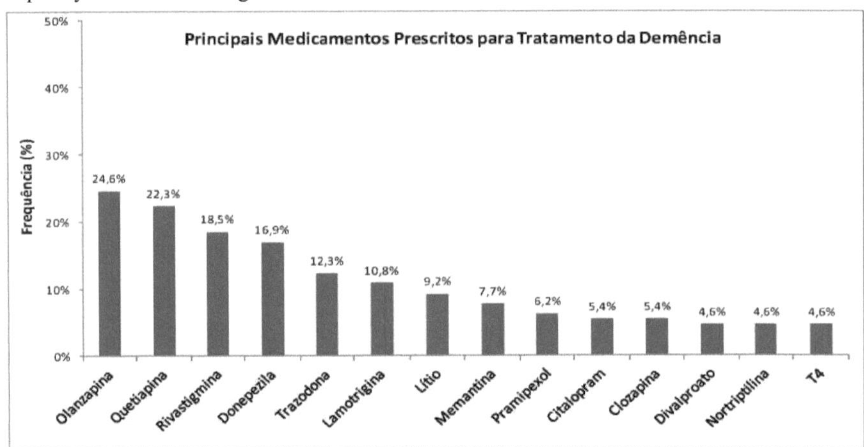

Figure 1: Main drugs prescribed in the treatment of dementia and concomitant bipolar disorder

4.1. RESULTS AND DISCUSSION ON THE ASSOCIATION BETWEEN BIPOLAR AFFECTIVE DISORDER AND DEMENTIA

The analysis described in Table 7 was carried out in order to check whether dementia is associated with psychic comorbidities of mood disorders, i.e. we wanted to answer the question: are patients with a psychic comorbidity more prone to dementia than patients without that psychic comorbidity? Table 7 shows the incidence of dementia in the group without the comorbidity and the incidence of dementia in the group with the comorbidity, for the main psychological comorbidities analysed in this study. The chi-square test shows no significant difference between the incidence of dementia in the two groups for all comorbidities (p-value greater than 0.05 for all evaluations and consequently odds ratios not significantly different from 1, with a confidence interval containing one). For example, dementia affects 72.1 per cent of patients without Bipolar I Disorder and 75.4 per cent of patients with Bipolar I Disorder, there is no significant difference between these proportions (p-value=0.666), there is no significantly increased chance of Bipolar I Disorder sufferers having dementia, and the confidence interval (CI) of the odds ratio contains the value 1.

Table 7: Association between dementia and the main psychological comorbidities of mood disorders.

Comorbidity Psychic	Not diagnosed and has dementia		Presents the diagnosis and has dementia		P.- test value X^2	OR	OR CI
Dementia and TBI	49/68	72,1%	46/61	75,4%	0,666	1,2	0,5-2,6
Dementia and Mixed BAD	62/80	77,5%	34/50	68,0%	0,230	0,6	0,3-1,4
Dementia and TBVI	65/185	76,5%	31/45	68,9%	0,349	0,7	0,3-1,5
Dementia and TBII	77/106	72,6%	19/24	79,2%	0,511	1,4	0,5-4,2

Fisher's exact test

The analysis described in Table 8 is intended to check whether not treating the psychological comorbidities of mood disorders increases the chance of the patient being diagnosed with specific types of dementia or some syndrome. Table 8 shows the incidence of the type of dementia in the subgroup of patients who did not treat psychological comorbidities and the incidence of the types of dementia in the subgroup of patients who did treat psychological comorbidities. The chi-square test showed no significant difference between the incidence of types of dementia in the subgroups of patients who treated and did not treat their comorbidities (p-value greater than 0.05 and OR not significant, OR CI containing the value 1 for all evaluations).

Table 8: Association between non-treatment/treatment of mood disorder comorbidities and types of dementia.

Type of Dementia	Did not treat comorbidity psychic (n=72)		Treated comorbidity Psychic (n–58)		P-value	OR	OR CI
Tabe Alzheimer's	20	27,8%	10	17,2%	0,156	0,5	0,2-1,3
Tab and Vascular	12	16,7%	16	27,6%	0,132	1,9	0,8-4,4
Tab and Frontotemporal	23	31,9	16	27,6	0,590	0,8	0,4-1,7
Tab and Corticobasal	25	34,7%	20	34,5%	0,977	0,99	0,5-2,0
Tabs and Lewy Bodies	7	9,7%	6	10,3%	0,906	1,1	0,3-3,9

In the same vein, a recent study points to results corroborating the thesis that bipolar disorder is a disease associated with accelerated ageing (Yang *et al.*, 2018).

4.2. TREATMENT RESULTS AND DISCUSSION

In a global analysis, the improvement of 71 patients was assessed. Of these 71 patients, 17 patients (23.9%) showed no improvement with treatment, 52 patients (73.2%) showed partial improvement and only two patients (2.8%) showed total improvement. Patient improvement was found to be independent of the patient's sex (p-value=0.759 from the chi-squared test), independent of whether or not they had previously treated their psychological comorbidity (p-value=0.443 from the chi-squared test), nor was it associated with the patient's age (p-value=0.943 from the Mann-Whitney test), nor with the patient's schooling (p-value=0.080 from the Mann-Whitney test), nor was it associated with the amount of medication used (p-value=0.943 from the Mann-Whitney test).

value=0.170 of the Mann-Whitney test), nor is it associated with the total number of crises (p-value=0.076 of the Mann-Whitney test).

Table 9 shows that, in terms of length of bipolar disorder, the results show that patient improvement is associated with length of psychological comorbidity. Patients who did not improve had an average of 16.4 years of psychological comorbidity, with a median of 7.5 years. Patients who showed some improvement had significantly longer psychological comorbidity, on average 26.2 years. This finding calls for some reflection. The patient with the longest comorbidity is no more protected from dementia than the patient with the shortest comorbidity, since psychic comorbidities are organic factors in the worsening and outcome of dementia. However, it is possible to assume that patients with comorbidities for a longer period of time start treatment for mood disorders earlier, which helps them from the onset of dementia, due to preventive behaviour (KIM, 2016; KIRSHENBON, 2017; FORLENZA, 2013 GOODMAN, 2015).

Table 9: Main statistics for the duration of psychological comorbidity in the group of patients who did not improve with treatment and the group of patients who showed some improvement.

	Time of psychiatric comorbidity					
Subgroup	**Average**	**Median**	**Minimum**	**Maximum**	**D.P**	**c.v**
No improvement	16,4	7,5	2,0	60,0	17,5	1,01
Partial or Total Improvement	26,2	20,0	0,5	70,0	18,0	0,69

Table 10 shows the frequency distributions of improvement by clinical condition, compared with the improvement of patients without the clinical condition. Among those with dementia syndrome and bipolar disorder with a predominance of manic crises, only 33.3 per cent showed any improvement, a significantly lower proportion than the proportion of improvement in patients with dementia syndrome and bipolar disorder without manic crises, 77.9 per cent (p-value=0.026 from Fisher's Exact test).

The results also made it possible to discuss whether the length of time of bipolar disorder and the number of crises interfere with dementia progression, as they showed that of the patients with dementia syndrome who had bipolar disorder predominantly in the manic phase, only 33.3 per cent showed any improvement in the dementia phase, a significantly lower proportion than the proportion of improvement in those who did not have mania syndrome, 77.9 per cent (BABA, 2016).

In this way, the manic state of bipolar disorder was considerably an aggravating factor in the treatment of patients with dementia. In this sense, it was found that the "type" of crisis, "mania", affects the outcome or dementia treatment more negatively than bipolar patients with a predominance of "depressive", hypomanic or cyclothymic crises.

Table 10: Frequencies of improvement by clinical condition, compared with the improvement of patients without the clinical condition

Clinical picture	**It gets better**	**Not shown the clinical picture**		**Features the clinical picture**		**p-value****
Dementia syndrome and bipolar disorder without specific crises	None	8	50,0%	9	16,4%	
	Partial	8	50,0%	44	80,0%	**0,006**
	Total	0	0,0%	2	3,6%	
Dementia syndrome and bipolar disorder with seizures depression	None	11	25,0	6	22,2%	
	Partial	32	72,7%	20	74,1%	0,790
	Total	1	2,3%	1	3,7%	
Dementia Syndrome and Bipolar Disorder with Cyclothymia	None	17	27,9%	0	0,0%	
	Partial	42	68,9%	10	100,0%	0,104*
	Total	2	3,3%	0	0,0%	
Dementia Syndrome and Bipolar Disorder with Syndrome extrapyramidal	None	14	23,3%	3	27,3%	
	Partial	44	73,3%	8	72,7%	0,718*
	Total	2	3,3%	0	0,0%	
Dementia Syndrome and Bipolar Disorder with other Psychiatric Syndromes	None	13	21,3%	4	40,0%	
	Partial	46	75,4%	6	60,0%	nc
	Total	2	3,3%	0	0,0%	
Dementia Syndrome and Bipolar disorder with attacks of hypomania.	None	15	24,2%	2	22,2%	
	Partial	46	74,2%	6	66,7%	1,000*
	Total	1	1,6%	1	11,1%	
Dementia Syndrome and Bipolar Disorder with bouts of Mania	None	13	20,0%	4	66,7%	
	Partial	50	76,9%	2	33,3%	**0,026***
	Total	2	1,0%	0	0,0%	

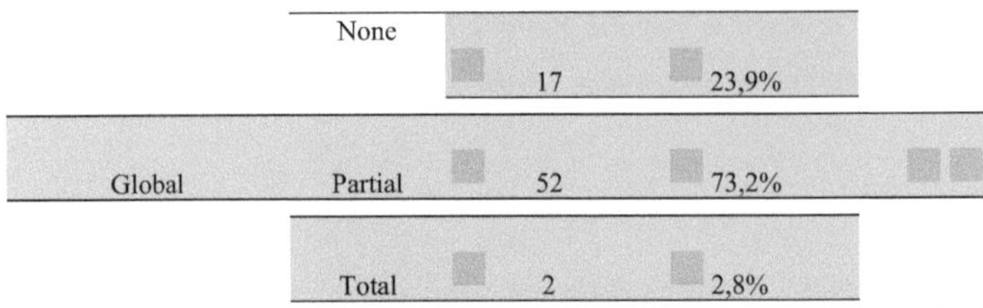

	None	17	23,9%
Global	Partial	52	73,2%
	Total	2	2,8%

1 * The tests were carried out considering two classifications "No improvement" and "Some improvement" (partial improvement or total improvement) *Fisher's Exact Test

The impact of lithium compared to other mood stabilisers was investigated. Only 12 patients who took lithium had their improvement assessed. Of these 12 patients, 1 (8.3%) had total improvement, 8 (66.7%) had partial improvement, and 3 patients (25.0%) had no improvement. In the group that used other drugs, these percentages were 1.7%, 74.6% and 23.7%, respectively. The chi-squared test showed no significant difference between these proportions.

As for the question about the difference between the impact of lithium when compared to other mood stabilisers, the results show that it is not significantly different from the effect of the other drugs evaluated in the patient's treatment. However, there is still a debate about the impact of lithium when compared to other mood stabilisers[1] in terms of neuroprotection, especially since different studies have found a reduction in the risk of dementia in subjects with bipolar affective disorder using lithium (MOTA DE FREITAS, 2016; TSAI, 2016; RIBAKOWSK, 2016).

Table 11 and Figure 2 analyse the improvement of patients by drug used for treatment, considering only the main drugs used. Only the Lamotrigine, Quetiapine and Lithium treatments have frequencies of patients with total improvement. The least inefficient treatments are those with Lamotrigine and Donepezil, as they have the lowest proportions of patients who showed no improvement.

Table 11: Analysis of Patient Improvement, by drug used for treatment.

Treatment	It gets better	Frequency
Olanzapine	None	316,7%
	Partial	1583 ,3%
	Total	00,0%
Quetiapine	None	316,7%
	Partial	1372 ,2%
	Total	211,1%
	None	213,3%

Rivas	Partial	1386	,7%
	Total		00,0%
	None		18,3%
Donepezil	Partial	1191	,7%
	Total		00,0%
	None		330,3%
Trazodone	Partial	770	,0%
	Total		00,0%
	None		18,3%
Lamotrigine	Partial	1083	,3%
	Total		18,3%
	None	3	25,0%
Lithium	Partial	8	66,7%
	Total	1	8,3%
	None	17	23,9%
Global	Partial	52	73,2%
	Total	2	2,8%

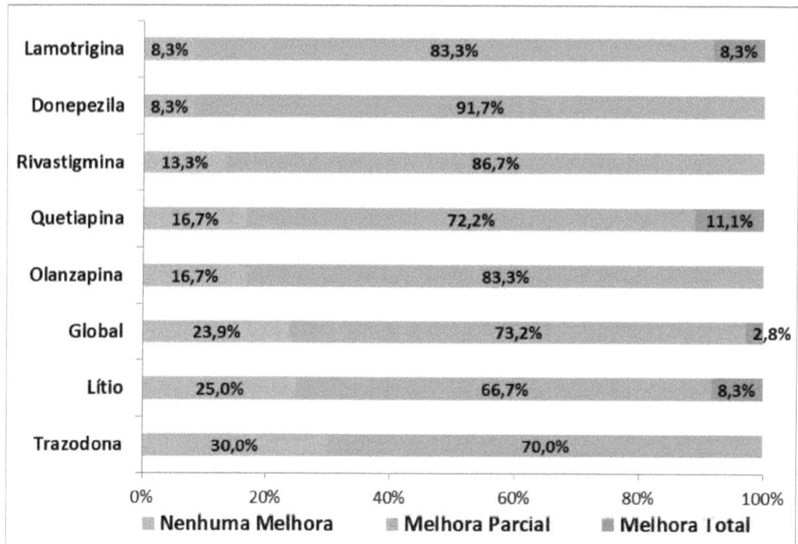

Figure 2: Analysis of Patient Improvement, by drug prescribed for treatment.

The most commonly used drugs in the treatment of the sample evaluated were Olanzapine (11.5% of the sample and 33.3% of those who used some medication) and Quetiapine (10.8% of the sample, 31.3% of those who used some medication). Lithium was the third main medication used for mood stabilisation, being used by 8.5% of the sample, or 24.4% of those using some medication. As can be seen, the atypical antipsychotic quetiapine and the antipsychotic olanzapine were the most commonly used in the treatment of the population studied, (OSBORNE, 2016; SUTHERLAND, 2015).

Psychosis is one of the most common conditions in the lives of older people, with dementia being a contributing factor. As such, antipsychotic drugs have been shown to be effective in managing psychosis associated with dementia (SEMLA *et al*, 2017).

CHAPTER 6

CONCLUSION

The conclusion is that there is no significant difference between the age of male and female patients; that there is no significant difference between the schooling of male and female patients; that in the population of patients with dementia and bipolar affective disorder, there is a significant predominance of women; that the treatment or non-treatment of psychic comorbidity is not associated with the patient's sex; that the treatment or non-treatment of psychic comorbidity is not associated with the patient's schooling; that the treatment or non-treatment of comorbidity is not associated with the age at which the comorbidity was discovered and that the treatment or non-treatment of comorbidity is associated with the time between the comorbidity and inclusion. Patients who did not treat their comorbidities had the comorbidity for longer than patients who treated the comorbidity.

We concluded that the treatment or non-treatment of the comorbidity is not associated with the number of seizures, because the number of seizures in the treatment group is not significantly different from the number of seizures in the group that does not treat the psychological comorbidity.

There was no significant difference between the age of onset of comorbidity in men and women (p-value=0.083).

There was no significant difference between the Years of Psychiatric Comorbidity until the inclusion of men and women in the sample (p-value = 0.039), i.e. the length of comorbidity was not associated with the patient's sex.

There was no significant difference between the number of seizures in men and women (p-value=0.992).

There was no significant difference between the number of drugs taken by men and women (p-value=0.951).

Dementia is not particularly associated with a specific type of bipolar affective disorder, but can prevail indistinctly, to varying degrees.

It is concluded that the effect of lithium is not significantly different from the effect of other drugs in improving the patient's condition. The use of lithium has shown preventive efficacy for the outcome of dementia according to other studies, but in this particular study it was not superior to other mood stabilisers during the treatment of patients with dementia and mood disorders.

The number of seizures due to bipolar disorder did not affect the improvement of patients with dementia afterwards. In this study, there was no evidence of a proportional link between bipolar disorder crises and a worse dementia prognosis.

With regard to the "type of crisis", it was clear that bipolar patients with a prevalence of manic crises had a worse recovery in dementia treatment than the others. In other words, the "type of crisis" variable had more influence than the "duration of crises" or "number of crises" variables.

REFERENCES

AKISKAL, H. S.; PINTO, O. The evolving bipolar spectrum.Prototypes I, II, III, and IV. **Psychiatr Clin North Am**, v. 22, n. 3, p. 517-34, vii, Sep 1999

ALMEIDA OP *et al.* Risk of dementia and death in community-dwelling older men with bipolar disorder. **Br J Psychiatry**.2016.

AZORIN, J. M.*et al.*Late-onset bipolar illness: the geriatric bipolar type VI. **CNS Neurosci Ther**, v. 18, n. 3, p. 208-13, Mar 2012.

BABAH. Depression and Bipolar Disorder: Risk Factors and Potential Prevention of Developing Dementia. **Brain Nerve**.2016.

BAEZ S *et al*. Brain structural correlates of executive and social cognition profiles in behavioural variant frontotemporal dementia and elderly bipolar disorder.**Neuropsychologia**. 2017.

BLAZER D. Bipolar Disorder and Dementia: Weighing the Evidence. **Am J Geriatr Psychiatry**₂ _Apr;25(4):363-364. 2017.

CERAMI, C *et al*. From genotype to phenotype: two cases of genetic frontotemporal lobar degeneration with premorbid bipolar disorder. **J Alzheimer Dis**, v. 27, n. 4, p. 79-7, 2011

CAIXETA, L. Corticobasal Degeneration. In: (Ed.). Dementias. São Paulo Brazil: Lemos Editora, 2004. ch. 16, p.350. Frontotemporal dementia. In: (Ed.). Dementia: a multidisciplinary approach. São Paulo, SP: **Atheneu Ed**., 2006a. p.251.

History of dementia and dementia in history: concepts and trends. In: (Ed.). Dementia: a multidisciplinary approach. São Paulo, SP: **Atheneu Ed.**, 2006b. p.8.

. Dementia in Parkinson's disease. **Rev. Bras. Psiquiatria**. vol.30 no.4. São Paulo Dec. 2008 Epub Nov 24, 2008.

CAIXETA, L. Non-Alzheimer's dementias: frontotemporal focal dementias. Porto Alegre. **Ed. Art Med.** 2010.

. Alzheimer's Disease, Porto Alegre: **Artmed,** 2012 p. 97-113. Chap. 7.

. Frontotemporal dementia and other non-Alzheimer's dementias. Porto Alegre. **Ed. Art Med.** 2016.

DALGALARRONDO, P. Psychopathology of Mental Disorders. 2ª ed. Porto Alegre: **Artmed:** 2008.

DINIZ BS *et al.* History of Bipolar Disorder and the Risk of Dementia: A Systematic Review and Meta-Analysis. **Am J Geriatr Psychiatry**. 2017

FAVERO LP, BELFIORE, P, SILVA FL, CHAN BL Data analysis: multivariate modelling for decision-making. Rio de Janeiro: **Elsevier**. 2009.

FORLENZA OV *et al.* Cognitive impairment in late-life bipolar disorder is not associated with Alzheimer's disease pathological signature in the cerebrospinal fluid. **BipolarDisorder**. 2016.

GAMA CS, KUNZ M, MAGALHÃES PV, KAPCZINSKI F. Staging and neuroprogression in bipolar disorder: a systematic, review of the literature. **Rev Bras Psiquiatria,** v. 35, n. 1, p. 70-74, Feb 2013.

GOODMAN C *et al.* End of life care interventions for people with dementia in care homes: addressing uncertainty within a framework for service delivery and evaluation. **BMC Palliat Care**,2015.

KESSING, L V; NILSSON, F M. Increased risk of developing dementia in patients with major affective disorders compared to patients with other medical illnesses. **J Affect Disorder**, v. 73, n. 3, p. 261-9, Feb 2003.

KIRSHENBOM D *et al.* Older Age, Comorbid Illnesses, and Injury Severity Affect Immediate Outcome in Elderly Trauma Patients. **J Emerg Trauma Shock,** Jul- Sep;10(3):146-150. 2017.

KIM HK *et al.* Neuropathological relationship between major depression and dementia: A hypothetical model and review. **Prog Neuropsychopharmacol Biol Psychiatry,** Jul- Sep;10(3):146-150. 2016.

KOTZIAN B, PASSOS I C, KAPCZINSKI F. Longitudinal course of bipolar disorder. **Revista Debates em Psiquiatria** v. 6, n. 5, p. 6-8, Sep/Oct. 2016.

MAGALHÃES PV, KAPCZINSKI F. Staging and neuroprogression in bipolar disorder: a systematic, review of the literature. **Rev Bras Psiquiatria,** 2013.

MEDRONHO RA. Epidemiology. São Paulo. **Atheneu Publishing House**.2009.

MOTA DE FREITAS D. Lithium in Medicine: Mechanisms of Action. **Met lons Life Sei.** 2016.

NG, B *et al*. A case series on the hypothesised connection between dementia and bipolar spectrum disorders: bipolar type VI? **J Affeet Disorder**, v. 107, n. 1-3, p. 307-15, Apr 2008.

OSBORNE V. Utilisation of extended release quetiapine (Seroquel XL™): Results from an observational cohort study in England. **Eur Psyehiatry,** Mar;33:61-67.2016.

PAPAZACHARIAS A, *et al*. Disorder and Frontotemporal Dementia: An Intriguing Association. **J Alzheimers Dis,** 55(3):973-979. 2017.

PICCINNI A, *et al*. Bipolar Disorder and dementia: a close link. **Clinieal Neuropsyehiatry,** 12, 2, 27-36.2015.

RIBAKOWSK, JK Effect of Lithium on Neurocognitive Functioning. 13(8):887. 2016.

RISE IV, HARO JM, GJERVAN B. Clinical features, comorbidity, and cognitive impairment in elderly bipolar patients. **Neuropsyehiatry Dis Treat**. 2016.

RUBINO *et al* . Late onset bipolar disorder and frontotemporal dementia with mutation in progranulin gene: a case report. 2017.

SEMLA *et al.* Off-Label Prescribing of Second-Generation Antipsychotics to Elderly Veterans with Posttraumatic Stress Disorder and Dementia. **J Am Geriatr Soc,** Aug;65(8):1789-1795. 2017.

SILVA JR, G M N. "Bipolar disorder associated with dementia: typology, clinical correlations and pathophysiology". Goiânia, 2015. 86p. **Dissertation (Master's Degree in Health Sciences: Medicine - Psychiatry)**. Faculty of Medicine, Federal University of Goiás, Goiânia, 2015.

SUTHERLAND C, DUTHIE AC. Invited commentary on Lithium treatment and risk for dementia in adults with bipolar disorder.**Br J Psychiatry,** Jul;207(1):52-54. 2015.

TSAI *et al.* Effect of valproic acid on dementia onset in patients with bipolar disorder.**J. AffectDisord**, Sep 1;201:131-6. 2016.

VALIENGO *et al.* Disorders in the elderly: prevalence, functional impact, and management challenges. **Neuropsychiatric Disease and Treatment**. 2016.

VASCONCELOS-MORENO *et al.* Cognitive performance and psychosocial functioning in patients with bipolar disorder, unaffected siblings, and healthy controls. **Rev. Bras. Psiquiatria**, v. 38, n. 4, p. 275-280. 2016.

YANG, F *et al.* Further evidence of accelerated aging in bipolar disorder: focus on Gdf-15. **Translational neuroscience**, p. 17/21. 2018.

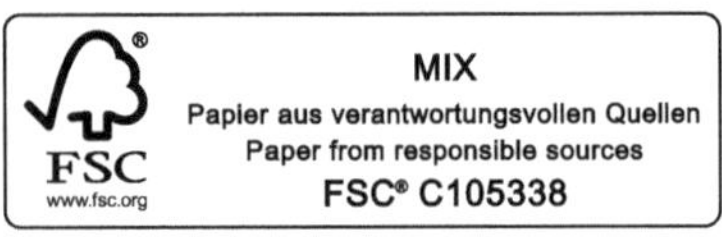

Printed by Books on Demand GmbH, Norderstedt / Germany